Seahorse's Magical Sun Sequences

by the same author

Frog's Breathtaking Speech
**How children (and frogs) can use yoga breathing
to deal with anxiety, anger and tension**
Michael Chissick
Illustrated by Sarah Peacock
ISBN 978 1 84819 091 7
eISBN 978 0 85701 074 2

Ladybird's Remarkable Relaxation
**How children (and frogs, dogs, flamingos and
dragons) can use yoga relaxation to help deal with
stress, grief, bullying and lack of confidence**
Michael Chissick
Illustrated by Sarah Peacock
ISBN 978 1 84819 146 4
eISBN 978 0 85701 112 1

of related interest

The Mouse's House
Children's Reflexology for Bedtime or Anytime
Susan Quayle
Illustrated by Melissa Muldoon
ISBN 978 1 84819 247 8
eISBN 978 0 85701 193 0

Connor the Conker and the Breezy Day
An Interactive Pilates Adventure
Rachel Lloyd
Foreword by Alan Watson
ISBN 978 1 84819 294 2
eISBN 978 0 85701 244 9

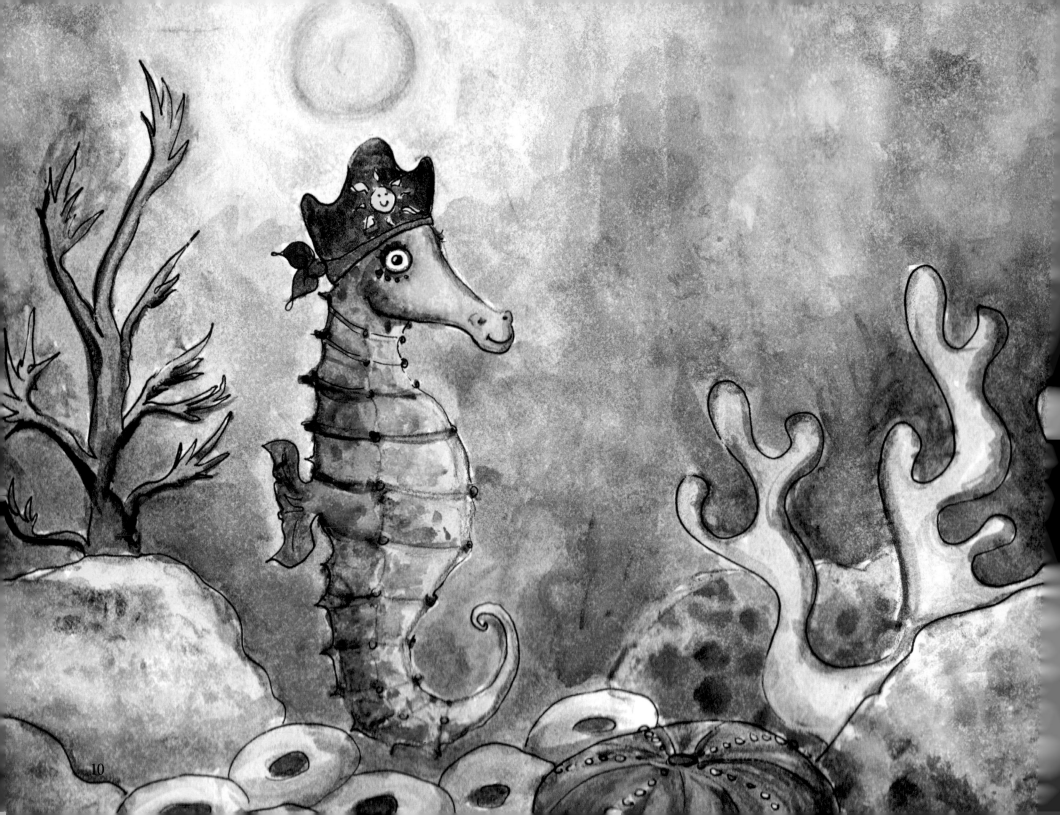

10

How to use this book

If you are a teacher in a school, the idea is that you choose the story (and therefore sequence) that is most appropriate to the children you are teaching so that everyone is included.

Similarly, if you are a parent, choose the story (and therefore sequence) that is most appropriate to your child or children's needs.

Whether you are a parent, educator or both, I suggest that you work on *one* story at a time. Read the story, or have your child or children read the story. When you come to the part when Seahorse teaches the Sun Sequence, jump in and do it three times. When you come to the part when one of the characters is going to lead, encourage one of the children or your child to lead. Again, I suggest that you work on the same chapter for a while to make sure that the sequence is well and truly learnt before you move on.

The posters of each sequence show you how to practise the individual postures. Simply copy what you see. They are straightforward and simple. Children's yoga is not about perfection in the posture. You'll forgive me if I shout that again loudly from the rooftops: *Children's yoga is not about perfection in the posture.*

Who is *Seahorse* for?

The *Seahorse* stories are aimed at children from 3–11 years old. However, stories like this defy age. The sequences themselves are suitable for children from 3–11 years and beyond, into adulthood. *Seahorse* is also a teaching resource for primary and elementary school teachers, head teachers, teaching assistants and people in the field of special needs who may have little or no knowledge of yoga. *Seahorse* is a *must-have* for children's yoga teachers, saving them hours of planning.

This yoga storybook is also for parents who are looking for a fun and engaging story to teach their children yoga and help them cope with issues that include inflexibility, self-esteem, disabilities and the complex sensory issues that come with autism.

The benefits of Sun Sequences for children

The Sun Sequence has been the most engaging activity in my yoga lessons since I began to teach yoga to children. Apart from the fact that children love them, sequences are highly effective in children's lessons for several reasons:

- Children enjoy the security of the structure that sequences bring – they feel more secure knowing what is coming next.

- Sequences demand concentration and co-ordination.

- They provide opportunities for children to step up and lead the class.

- Children enjoy the flowing body movement.

- It is a more invigorating way to practice yoga compared to isolated postures.

- Some children find sequences easy to remember and can teach them to friends and family members.

Also, sequences are:

- remarkably simple, fun and easy to learn

- easily adaptable for everyone

- usable practically anywhere

- genuinely yoga based.

Guidance for Teachers, Professionals and Parents

About this book

I wrote this book to give teachers, educators and parents the tools to enable *all* children to be included in the Sun Sequence, irrespective of any impairment.

The book contains five stories that each contain a specific sequence, reflecting the needs of four different groups of children.

The Starfish Brothers is suitable for children aged 3–5 years old in kindergarten, nursery, elementary or primary school. It is also suitable for older children, who may find other sequences too challenging at the moment.

Eel's Story is suitable for children in wheelchairs or children who find it difficult to stand.

Crab's Story is suitable for the majority of children on the Autism Spectrum.

Octopus's Story is suitable for older children (6–11 years old) who may find standing difficult or who may be going through a temporary problem, for example a broken leg.

The Starfish Brothers *Return* is suitable for the majority of 'able-bodied' children aged 6–11 years old.

Each story has the same format and storyline. This makes for good anticipation and reinforcement when children are practising their reading. The idea is that you dip into the story that most suits the needs of the children or child in front of you.

What is the Sun Sequence?

The Sun Sequence, also known as Sun Salutation or Salute to the Sun (Surya Namaskar), is one of the most popular and essential parts of any yoga lesson, whether children's or adult's. Put simply, it is a series of flowing yoga postures.

One of the objectives of the sequence is to move the spine in a variety of ways to increase flexibility. If you've tried it, you will know that it exercises the whole body. Some people use it as their wake-up morning routine; others as a bedtime solution to help sleep. If you are short of time, it can act as a whole session.

Sequences that are tried and tested

I have taught the children's Sun Sequence in every possible situation that you can imagine. That includes children with the most challenging and severe physical needs, children across the autism spectrum, children with intense emotional and behavioural needs, early years children and the whole range of mainstream primary. Over the years I have developed four sequences that will ensure that every child is included. Those four sequences have formed the basis of this book.

All four sequences have been tried, tested and developed in schools for nearly two decades – so you know they will work.

Contents

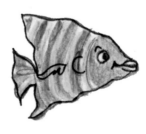

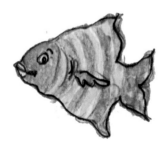

Acknowledgements

I would like to thank the head teachers who had the courage and belief to allow yoga in their schools as part of the curriculum. Thanks to them, Seahorse's Sun Sequence has grown and developed into an activity that has helped and continues to help hundreds of children become fitter and feel included in a physical activity where they may not have before.

In particular, I would like to express my huge gratitude to:

- Nick Heald, Head of Holdbrook Primary School, Waltham Cross, Hertfordshire

- Sarah Goldsmith, Head of Downfield Primary School, Cheshunt, Hertfordshire

- Stewart Harris and Veronica Armson, Head and Deputy Head at Phoenix School, Bow, East London.

I would also like to say an enormous thank you to all those class teachers, teaching assistants and learning support assistants who bend, stretch, squat and sing week in week out to make our yoga lessons fun and beneficial to the children that are lucky enough to be there; in particular, all the staff of Phoenix School, Woodcroft School, Holdbrook school and Downfield School.

Finally, thank you to all the children who regularly reach for the sun every week and hopefully will be reaching for the sun throughout their lives.

This book is dedicated to:

William Leighton Price,
a wonderful primary school teacher
who made such a difference to so many lives – *MC*

For my wonderful little boy, Albi – *SP*

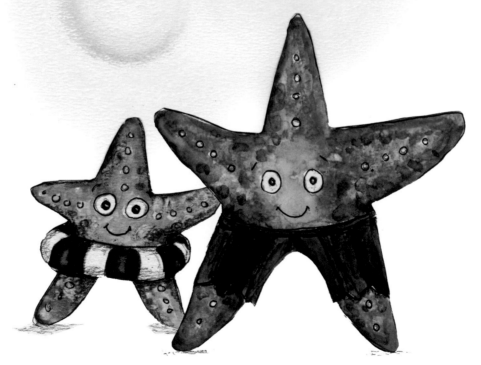

First published in 2016
by Singing Dragon
an imprint of Jessica Kingsley Publishers
73 Collier Street
London N1 9BE, UK
and
400 Market Street, Suite 400
Philadelphia, PA 19106, USA

www.singingdragon.com

Library of Congress Cataloging in Publication Data
A CIP catalog record for this book is available from the Library of Congress

British Library Cataloguing in Publication Data
A CIP catalogue record for this book is available from the British Library

ISBN 978 1 84819 283 6
eISBN 978 0 85701 230 2

Printed and bound in China

Seahorse's
MAGICAL
Sun Sequences

How all children (and sea creatures)
can use yoga to feel positive,
confident and completely included

Michael Chissick
Illustrated by Sarah Peacock

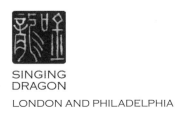

SINGING
DRAGON

LONDON AND PHILADELPHIA

Seahorse's Yoga
Sun Sequences

Seahorse glided easily in and out of the colourful coral.
Above her head a ball of golden sunshine glowed brightly,
lighting up the sea.

Seahorse was very happy. She thought to herself,
"Who can I help today?"

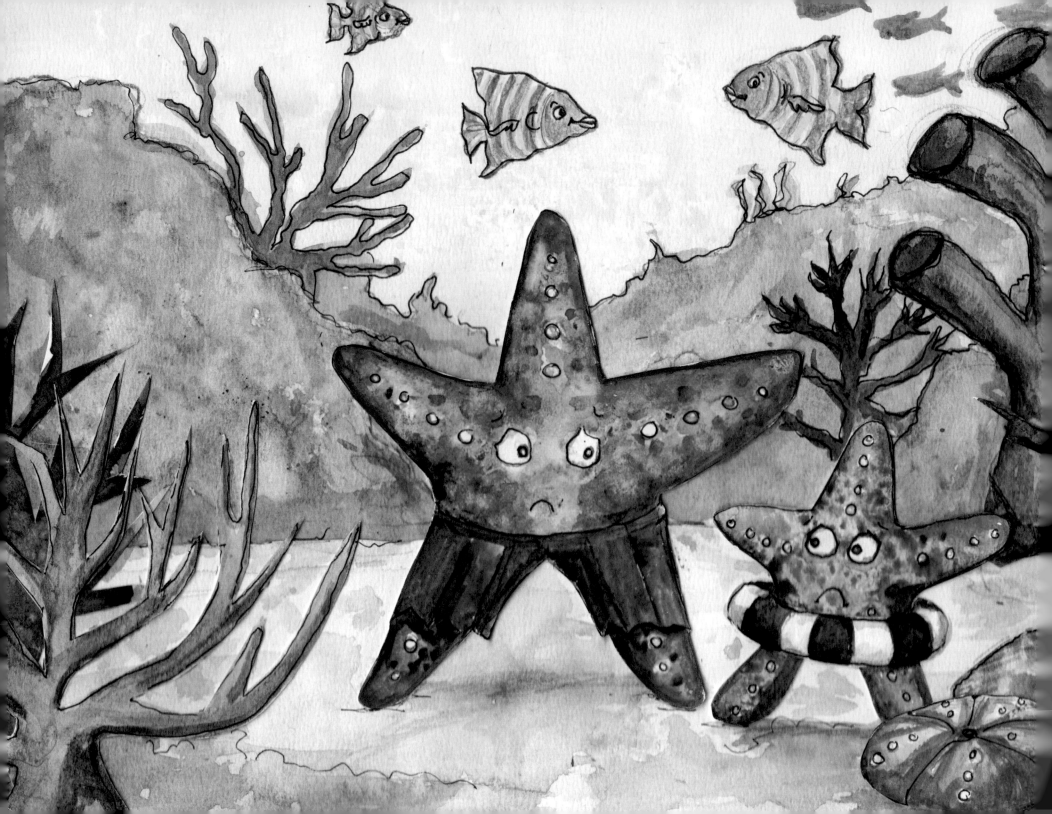

The Starfish Brothers

The Starfish Brothers, Toddler and Junior, creaked and moaned with each step as they dragged themselves across the sandy seabed.

"You're slower than the slowest water snail," said Seahorse. "What *is* the matter?" she asked.

"Our backs are stiff," said Toddler.

"Extremely stiff," added Junior. "So stiff we can only drag ourselves around like old wood from a shipwreck."

"We've tried all sorts of seaweed potions and jellyfish cures, but *nothing* helps," added Toddler.

"Everyone seems to be doing exciting things with their bodies on the coral reef except us," said Toddler. "We feel left out. We feel like shipwrecks. It's awful," said Junior.

"In that case I shall teach you the Sun Sequence," said Seahorse.

"What's that?" they asked.

"That's the reason I have a bright glow above my head, and it's great for making stiff backs flexible," said Seahorse. "I will teach it to you."

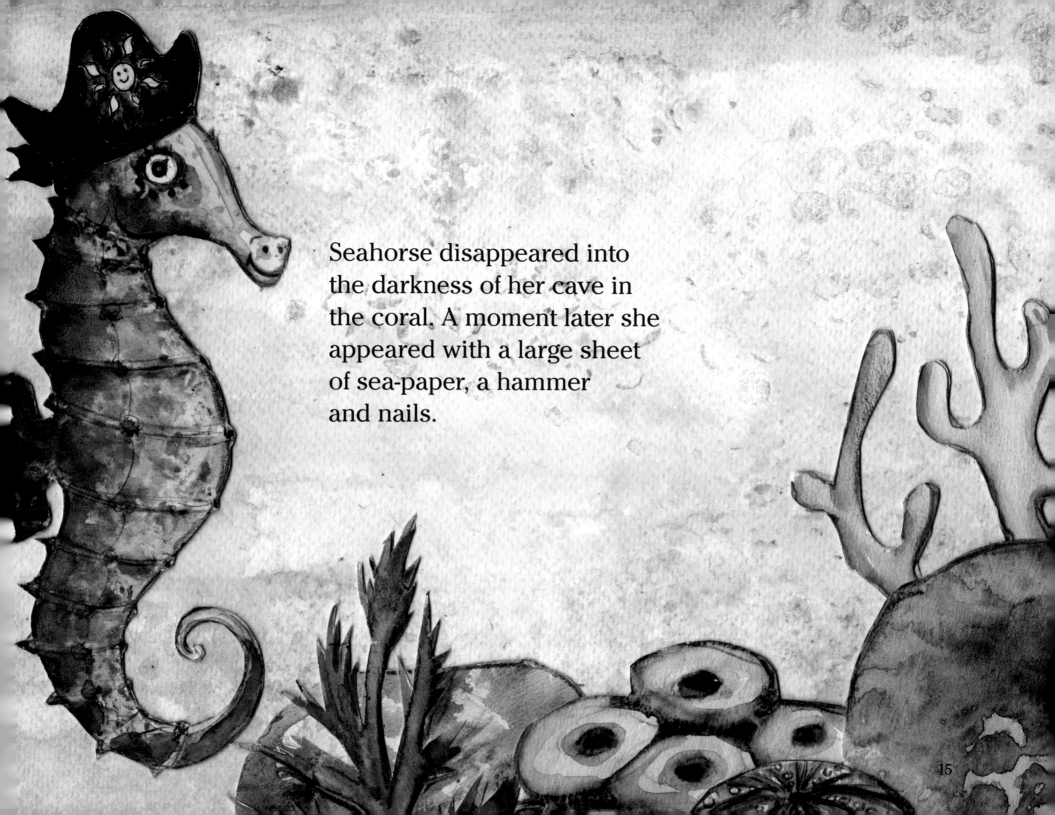

Seahorse disappeared into
the darkness of her cave in
the coral. A moment later she
appeared with a large sheet
of sea-paper, a hammer
and nails.

"This poster shows you how to do the Sun Sequence," she said. "I found it ages ago among some sunken treasure. Luckily it's made of sea-paper and cannot break into pieces."

Seahorse nailed the poster to a high rock.

"Here are all the moves," she said, pointing to the poster. "It is a human doing them. But that's OK. It shows us what to do. Let's do them together."

"But Seahorse, how? Look at the pictures. There is a lot of bending and we cannot bend with stiff backs," they said.

"Just go as far as you can. Do your best. Here we go. I'll say it and do it and you just copy. You'll soon get the hang of it. Ready?"

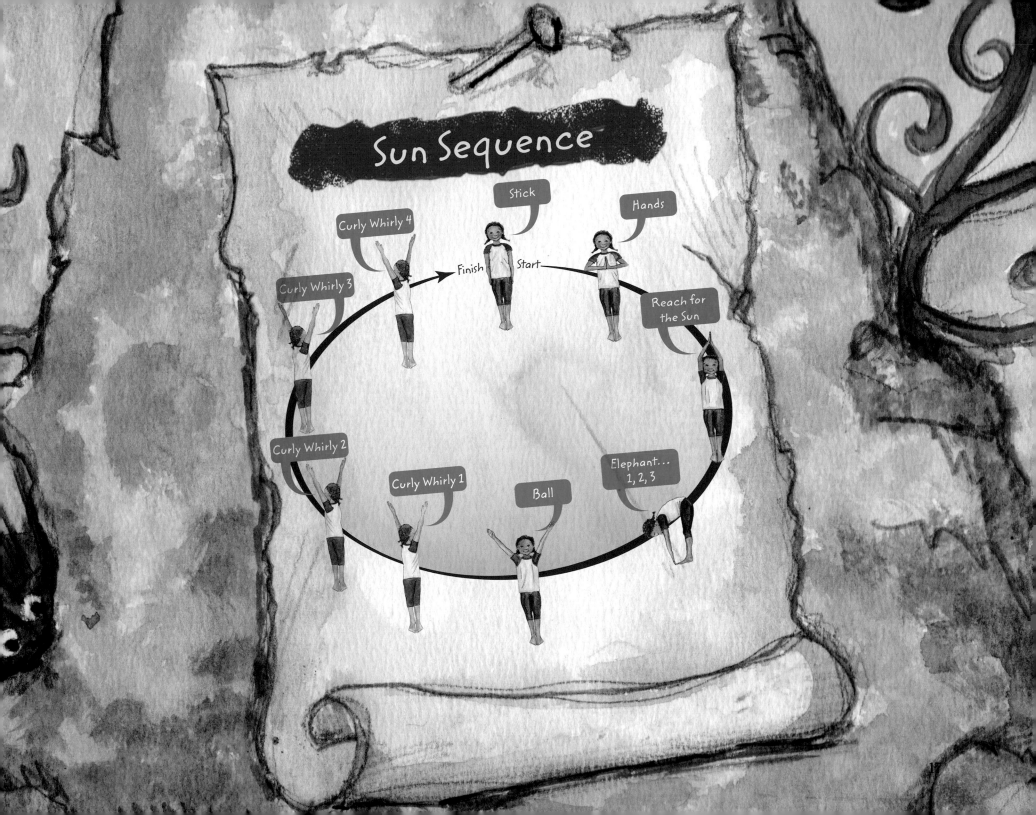

Toddler and Junior said and copied every move. Even though they were stiff, they were able to bend and twist. They were so happy. In fact, they were so happy they asked if they could do it again.

"Of course," said Seahorse. "Junior, would you like to lead?"

Junior stepped up, glanced at the paper nailed to the rock and called out the moves.

This time they both bent further forwards in Elephant, and they twisted further in Curly Whirly.

"It's not very often we see the Sun, living here among the coral, but if it wasn't for the Sun none of us would be here. So when we do the Sun Sequence

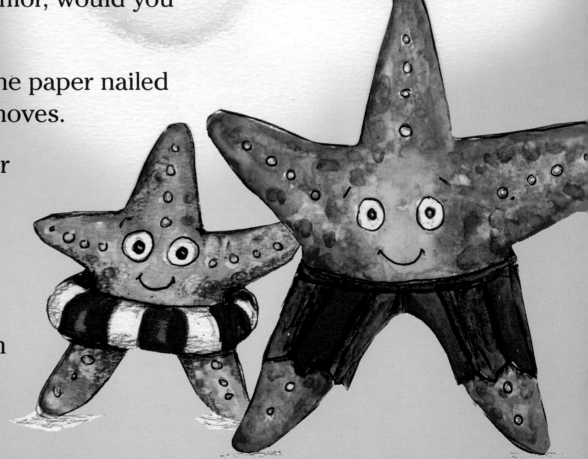

we can remind ourselves that the Sun is special and maybe a little bit magical," said Seahorse.

"Which is why," she continued, "when I think about the Sun Sequence, a bright glow appears above my head."

"Thank you and goodbye!" said the Starfish Brothers as they glided silently and easily across the seabed.

Seahorse watched them disappear over the horizon, until all that was left was a brilliant glow above their heads.

A wide smile swept across her face as she glided easily in and out of the coral. Seahorse was happy and ready to deal with whatever the sea-day had to bring. She thought to herself, "Who else can I help today?"

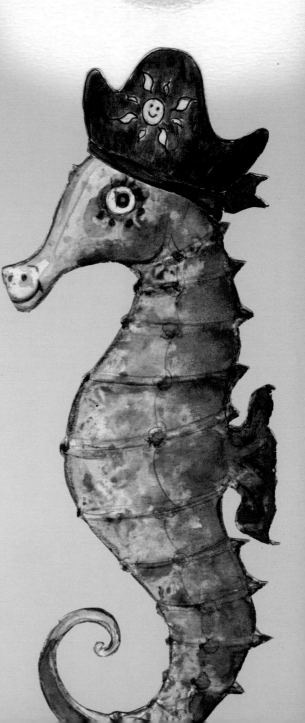

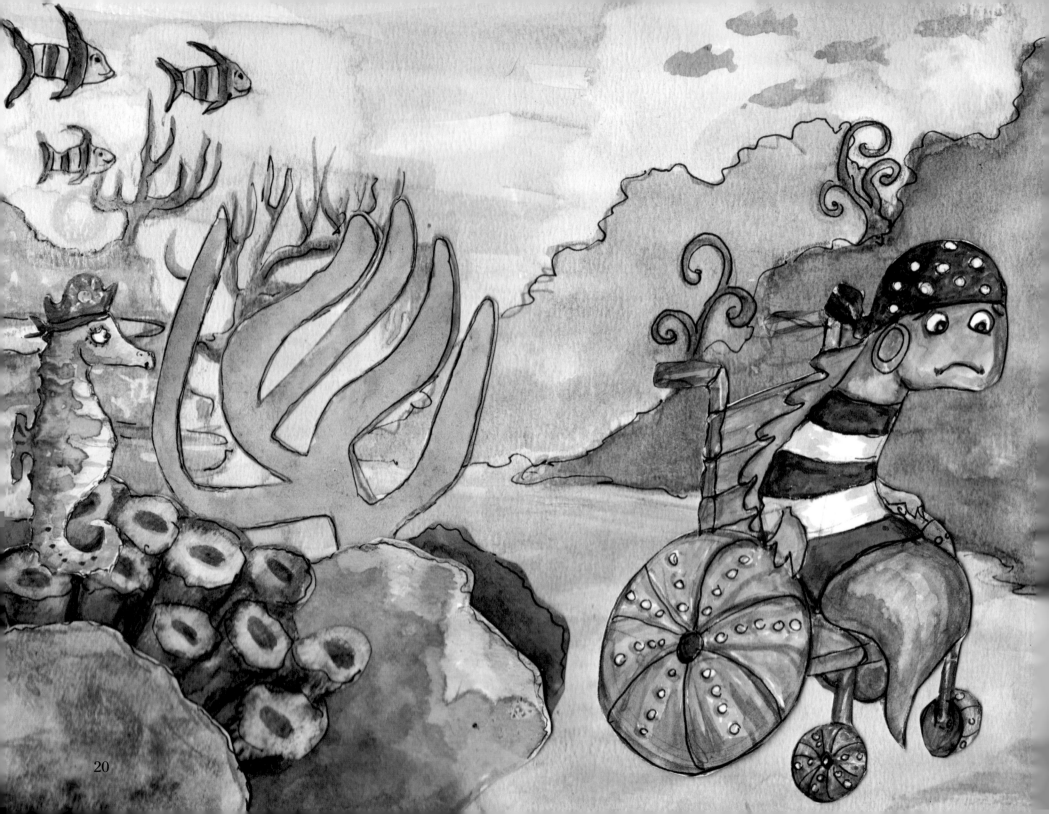

Eel

Eel sat sadly in his wheelchair.

Seahorse asked, "You look unhappy, Eel, what's the matter?"

"Being in a wheelchair means that there are lots of things I cannot do," said Eel. "I have forgotten what some of my body parts do. I feel that those parts of my body are useless. That makes me sad."

"In that case I shall teach you the Sun Sequence. You can do it in your wheelchair," said Seahorse.

"What's that?" asked Eel.

"That's the reason I have a bright glow above my head. It's great for Eels in wheelchairs because it helps you to know your body better," said Seahorse. "I will teach you how to do it."

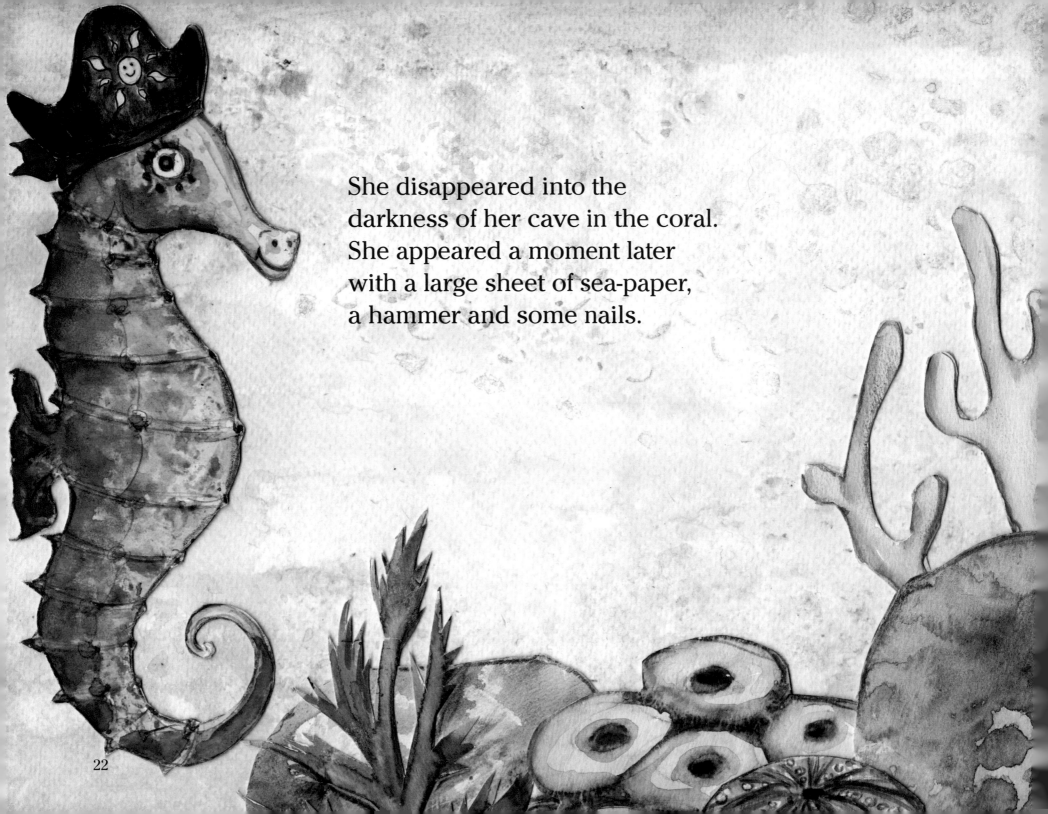

She disappeared into the
darkness of her cave in the coral.
She appeared a moment later
with a large sheet of sea-paper,
a hammer and some nails.

Seahorse nailed the poster to a high rock.

"This poster shows you how to do the Sun Sequence" Seahorse said. "I found it ages ago among sunken treasure. Luckily it is made of sea-paper and cannot dissolve."

"Here are all the moves," she said, pointing to the shabby poster. "It is a human doing them. But that's OK. It shows us what to do. Let's do them together."

"But Seahorse, I am in a wheelchair, how can I do the moves?" exclaimed Eel.

"No problem, Eel, this sequence is especially for Eels in wheelchairs." said Seahorse. "Just go as far as you can. Do your best. Here we go. I'll say it and do it and you just copy. You'll soon get the hang of it. Ready?"

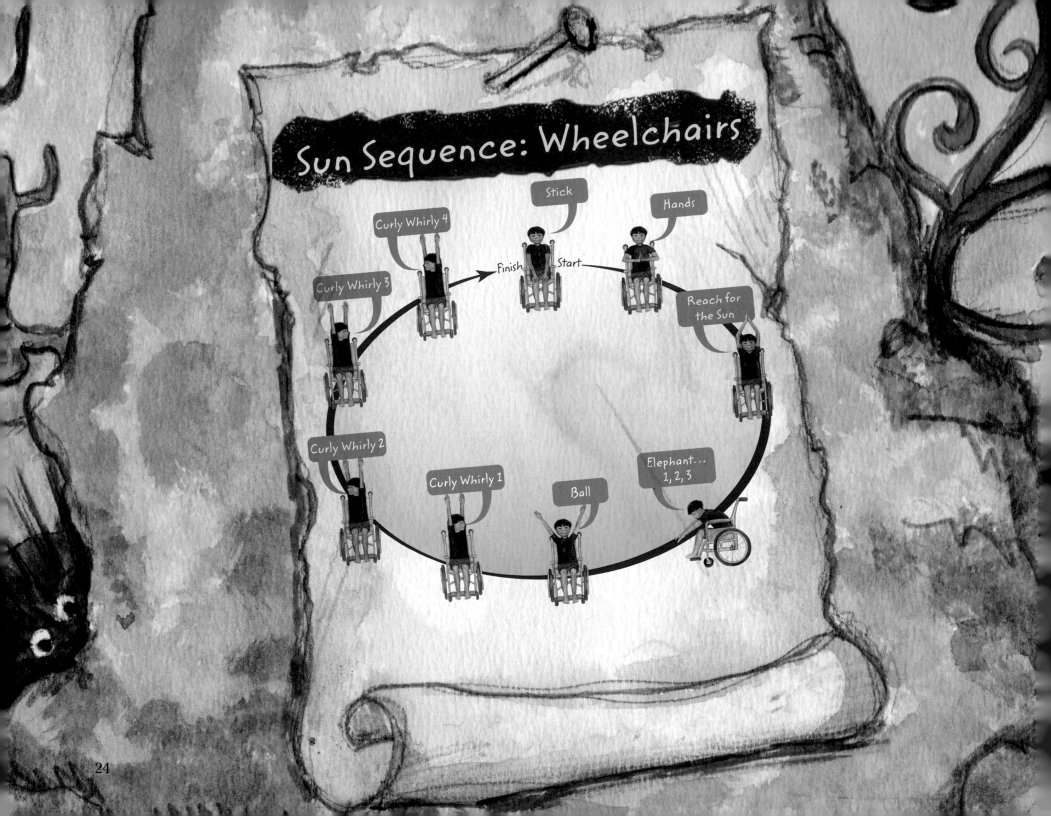

Eel said and copied every move. Even though he was in a wheelchair he could bend forwards in Elephant and twist sideways in Curly Whirly. He was very happy. He was so happy that he asked to do it again.

"Of course," said Seahorse. "Eel, would you like to lead this time?"

Eel wheeled himself over to the poster nailed to the rock. He was able to call out and do the moves. This time he bent a little further forward in Elephant and twisted even more in the Curly Whirly.

"It's not very often we see the Sun, living here among the coral, but if it wasn't for the Sun none of us would be here. So when we do the Sun Sequence we can remind ourselves that the Sun is special and maybe a little bit magical," said Seahorse.

"Which is why," she continued, "when I think about the Sun Sequence, a bright glow appears above my head."

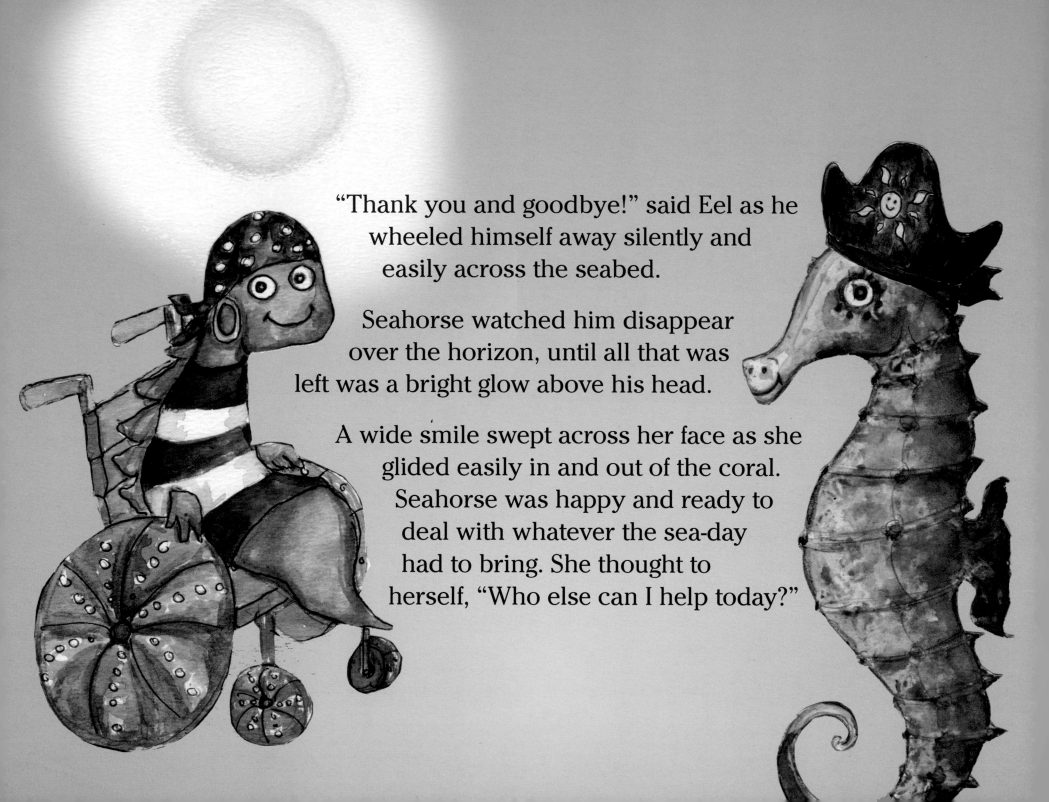

"Thank you and goodbye!" said Eel as he wheeled himself away silently and easily across the seabed.

Seahorse watched him disappear over the horizon, until all that was left was a bright glow above his head.

A wide smile swept across her face as she glided easily in and out of the coral. Seahorse was happy and ready to deal with whatever the sea-day had to bring. She thought to herself, "Who else can I help today?"

Crab

Crab had been hiding behind a rock. He had watched Seahorse teach Eel the Sun Sequence.

"I know you," said Seahorse, spotting Crab. "You are Crab. You don't speak. I've seen you around the coral. Did you see Eel doing the Sun Sequence?"

Crab nodded: "Yes."

"Would you like to do it?" Seahorse asked.

Crab shook his head: "No."

"Is that because you don't like moving?" Seahorse asked.

Crab nodded: "Yes."

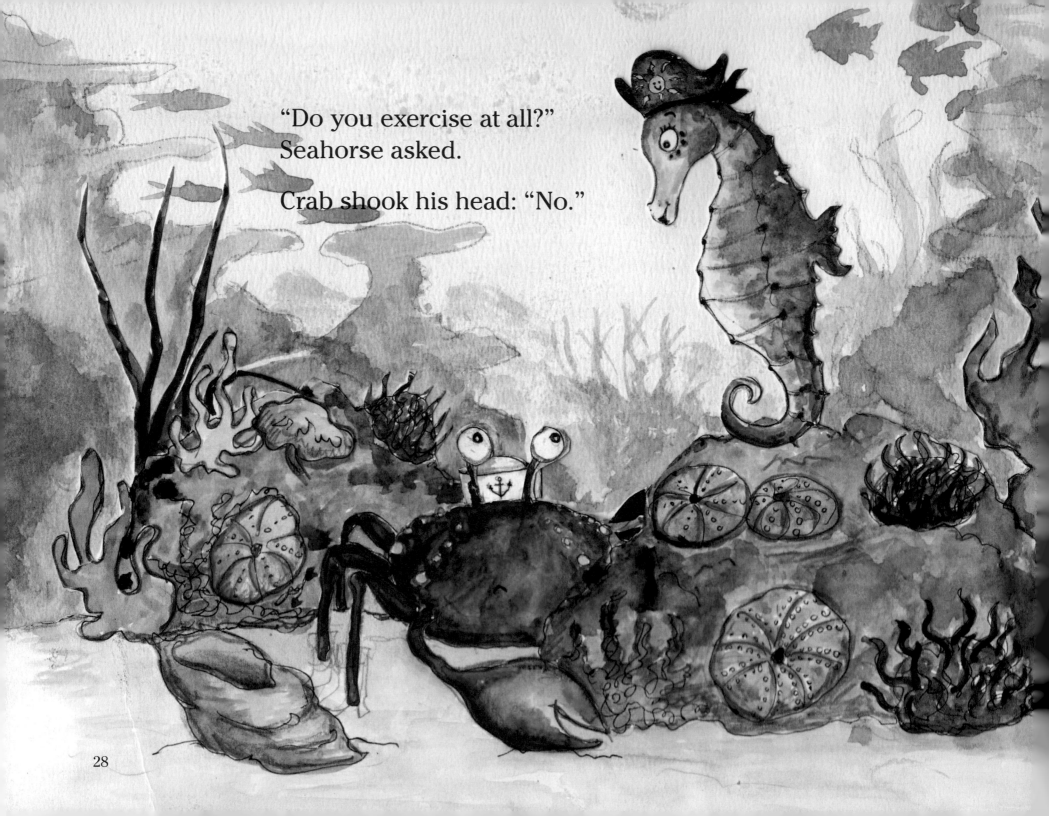

"Do you exercise at all?"
Seahorse asked.

Crab shook his head: "No."

28

"Is that because it is not fun for you?" Seahorse asked.

Crab nodded: "Yes."

"Crab," asked Seahorse, "do you like to do things in a strict order?"

Crab nodded: "Yes," with enthusiasm this time.

"Crab, if you like to do things in a strict order and in a fun way, then you will like the Sun Sequence."

Crab did not nod at all.

Seahorse said, "Will you be brave and let me teach you the Sun Sequence?"

Crab was very still for a moment. Then he nodded: "Yes."

Seahorse disappeared into the darkness of her cave in the coral. She appeared a moment later with a large sheet of sea-paper, a hammer and some nails.

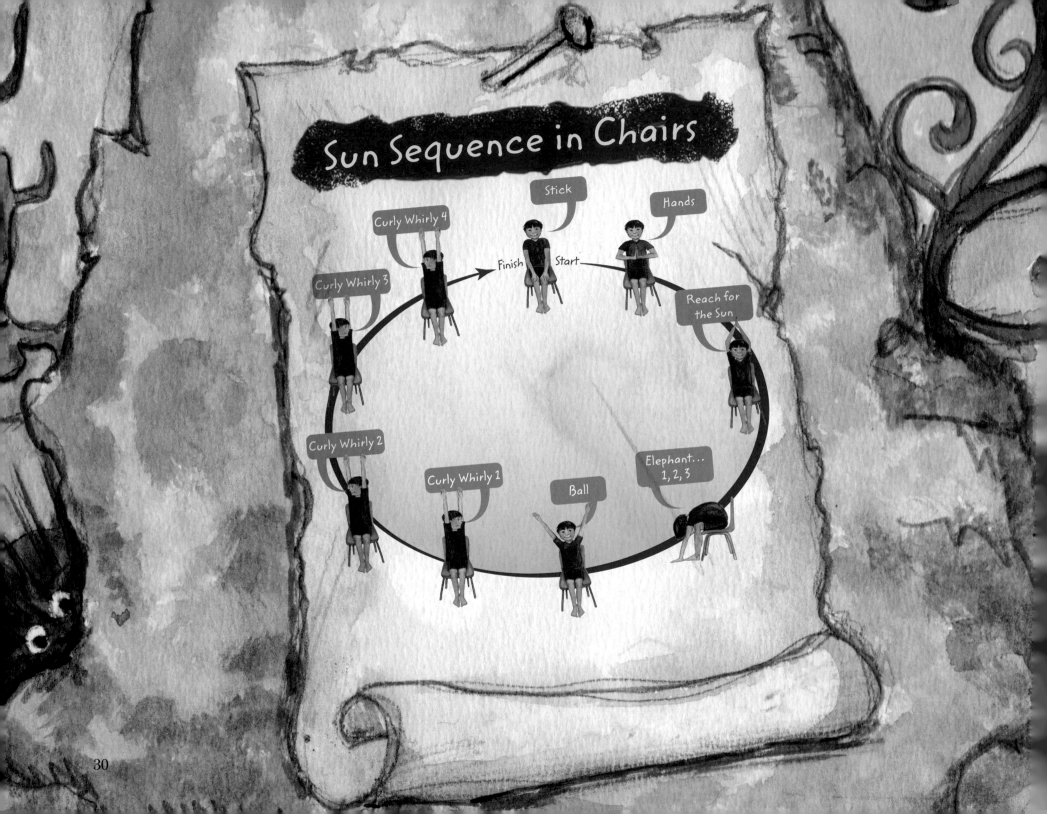

"This poster shows you how to do the Sun Sequence," Seahorse said. "I found it ages ago among sunken treasure. Luckily it is made of sea-paper and cannot dissolve."

Seahorse nailed the paper to a high rock.

"Here are all the moves," she said. "It is a human doing them. But that's OK. It shows us what to do. Let's do them together."

Crab looked lost.

"Are you overwhelmed in this space?" asked Seahorse.

Crab nodded: "Yes."

"Don't worry, Crab, you can do it on a chair. You'll feel safe in the chair and won't feel overwhelmed by the space around you," said Seahorse, fetching a chair from her cave. "And more good news, this sequence is especially for Crabs who do not like to move much or speak," said Seahorse. "Just go as far as you can. Do your best. Here we go. I'll say it and do it and you just copy. You'll soon get the hang of it. Ready?"

Crab nodded: "Yes."

Crab copied every move. And surprise, surprise, he said the names of the moves in a tiny voice. Crab looked very happy.

"You have a lovely voice," said Seahorse, "it's good to hear it. Would you like to do the sequence again?"

"Yes," said Crab in his tiny voice.

"How about you lead this time?" suggested Seahorse.

Crab walked over to the poster nailed to the rock. Using his tiny voice he was able to say and do the moves. This time he spoke a little louder.

He did not need to look at the poster to see what came next. He simply remembered. Crab had an excellent memory.

"It's not very often we see the Sun, living here among the coral, but if it wasn't for the Sun none of us would be here. So when we do the Sun Sequence we can remind ourselves that the Sun is special and maybe a little bit magical," said Seahorse.

"Which is why," she continued, "when I think about the Sun Sequence a bright glow appears above my head."

"Thank you and goodbye," said the Crab in his soft voice.

Crab sat happily on the chair, a bright glow above his head. He would rather sit on the chair now than hide behind the rock.

A wide smile swept across Seahorse's face as she glided easily in and out of the coral. Seahorse was happy and ready to deal with whatever the sea-day had to bring. She thought to herself, "Who else can I help today?"

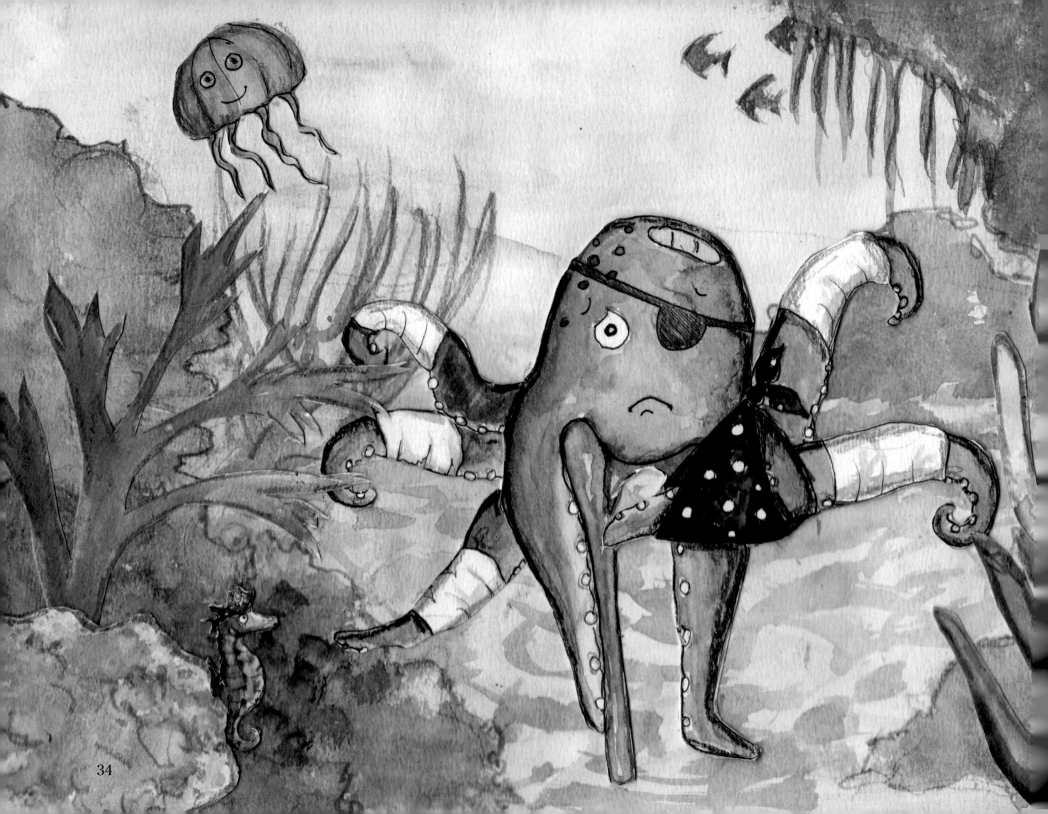

Octopus

Octopus leaned against the coral to catch his breath. It wasn't easy getting around in the sea on crutches. He was tired and fed up.

"What happened to you?" asked Seahorse when she spotted Octopus.

"I broke six legs competing in the pole vault in the Ocean Olympic Games," Octopus replied. "I was certain that I was clear of the bar when my pole snapped in two and I tumbled head over legs onto the judge. He was not pleased, and nor was I. Now I am fed up because I enjoy sports and competing. With six broken legs what can I win?"

"Octopus," said Seahorse, "I will teach you the Sitting Sun Sequence."

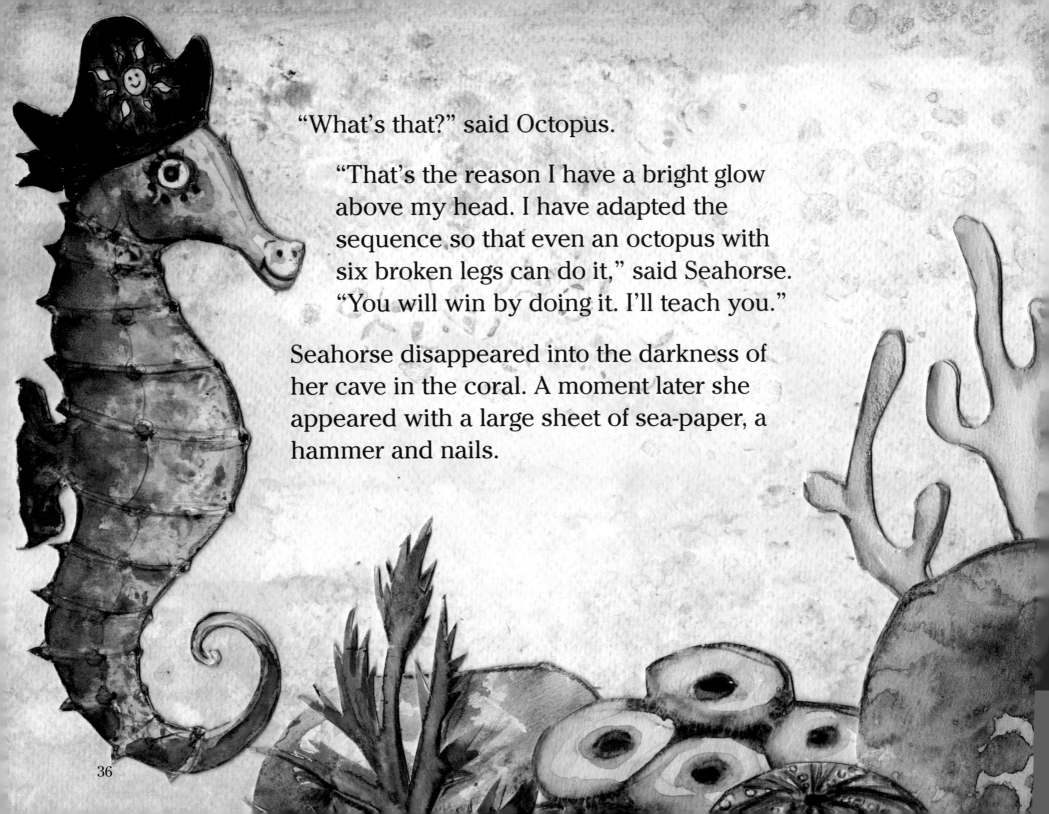

"What's that?" said Octopus.

"That's the reason I have a bright glow above my head. I have adapted the sequence so that even an octopus with six broken legs can do it," said Seahorse. "You will win by doing it. I'll teach you."

Seahorse disappeared into the darkness of her cave in the coral. A moment later she appeared with a large sheet of sea-paper, a hammer and nails.

"This poster shows you how to do the Sitting Sun Sequence," she said. "I found it ages ago among some sunken treasure. Luckily it's made of sea paper and cannot dissolve."

Seahorse nailed the poster to a high rock.

"Here are all the moves," she said. "It is a human doing them. But that's OK. It shows us what to do. Let's do them together."

"But Seahorse, how can I do anything physical in my condition?"

"Just go as far as you can. Do your best. Here we go. I'll say it and do it. You just copy. You'll soon get the hang of it. Ready?"

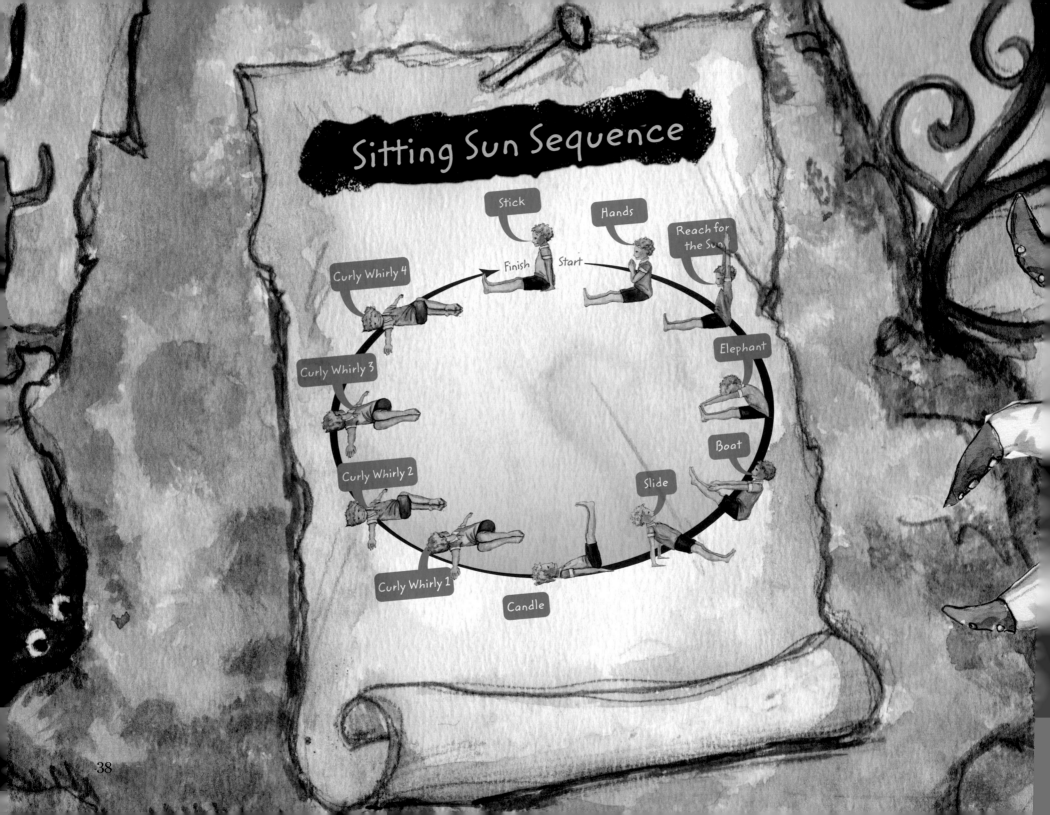

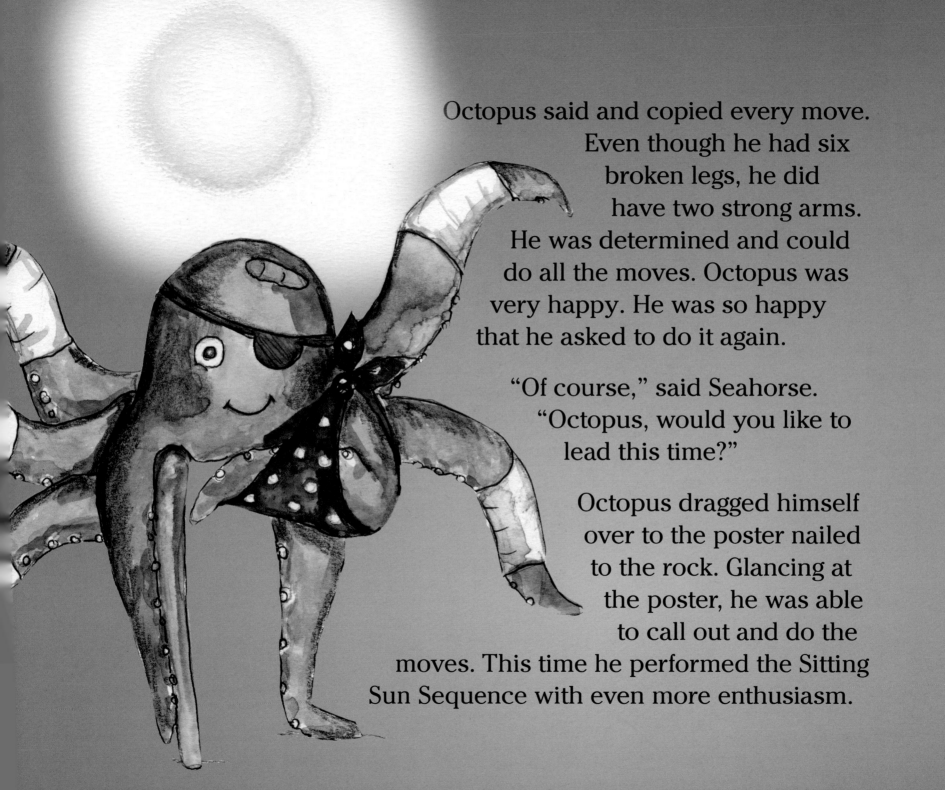

Octopus said and copied every move. Even though he had six broken legs, he did have two strong arms. He was determined and could do all the moves. Octopus was very happy. He was so happy that he asked to do it again.

"Of course," said Seahorse. "Octopus, would you like to lead this time?"

Octopus dragged himself over to the poster nailed to the rock. Glancing at the poster, he was able to call out and do the moves. This time he performed the Sitting Sun Sequence with even more enthusiasm.

"It's not very often we see the Sun, living here among the coral, but if it wasn't for the Sun none of us would be here. So when we do the Sun Sequence we can remind ourselves that the Sun is special and maybe a little bit magical," said Seahorse.

"Which is why," she continued, "when I think about the Sun Sequence a bright glow appears above my head."

"Thank you and goodbye!" said Octopus, as he sped away on his crutches.

Seahorse watched him disappear over the horizon, until all that was left was a bright glow above his head.

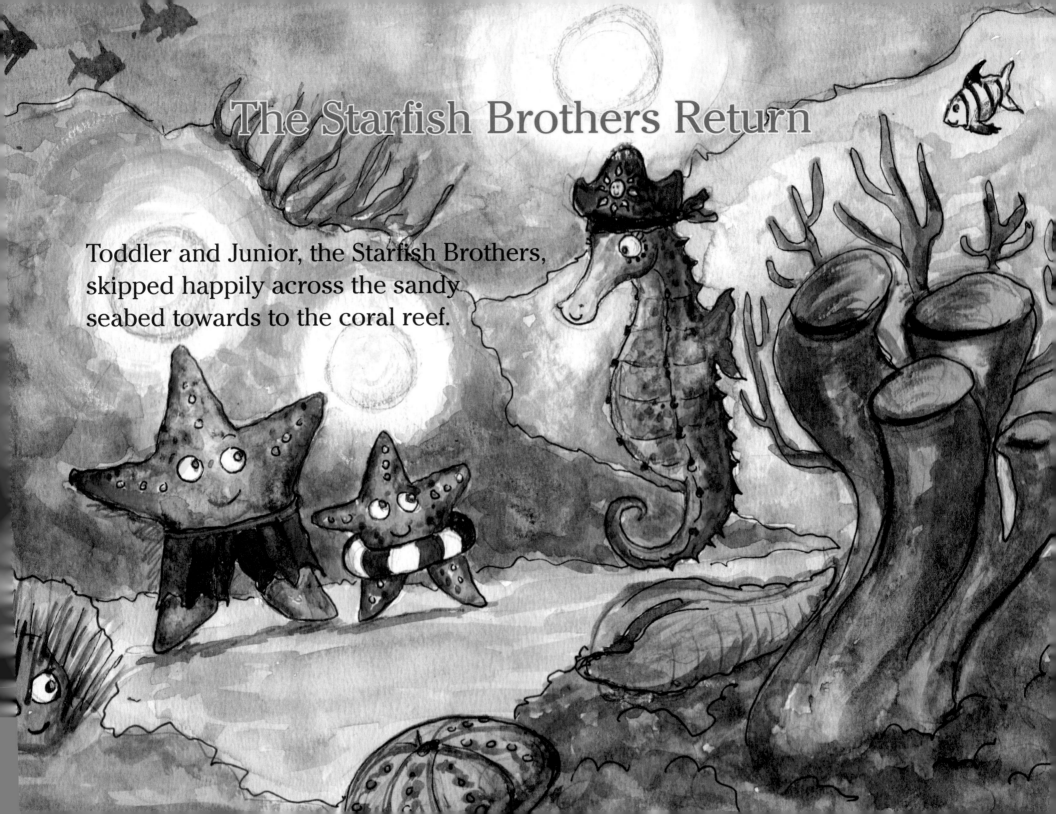

The Starfish Brothers Return

Toddler and Junior, the Starfish Brothers, skipped happily across the sandy seabed towards to the coral reef.

"Your movement is more graceful than a shark's," said Seahorse. "It's great to see you both again. I haven't seen you for six months. How are your stiff backs?"

"Our backs are no longer stiff, Seahorse. Because we practice the Sun Sequence every day, they are flexible," said the Starfish Brothers.

"Extremely flexible," added Junior, "which means that we do lots of exciting things around the coral and do not feel left out."

"That is very good news," said Seahorse. "Would you like to learn another Sun Sequence that is more challenging?"

"Yes please!" they replied.

"In that case, I shall teach you another Sun Sequence," Seahorse said.

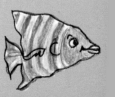

Seahorse disappeared into the darkness of her cave in the coral. A moment later she appeared with a large sheet of sea-paper, a hammer and nails.

"This poster shows you how to do the more challenging Sun Sequence," she said. "I found it ages ago among some sunken treasure with all the other Sun Sequences. Luckily it's made of sea-paper and cannot dissolve." Seahorse nailed the poster to a high rock.

"Here are all the moves," she said. "It is a human doing them. But that's OK. It shows us what to do. Let's do them together like we did last time."

"Look at the pictures," said the Starfish Brothers. "It looks more challenging. Do you think we can do it?"

"Just go as far as you can," replied Seahorse. "Do your best. Here we go. I'll say it and do it and you just copy. You'll soon get the hang of it. Ready?"

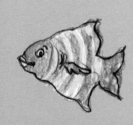

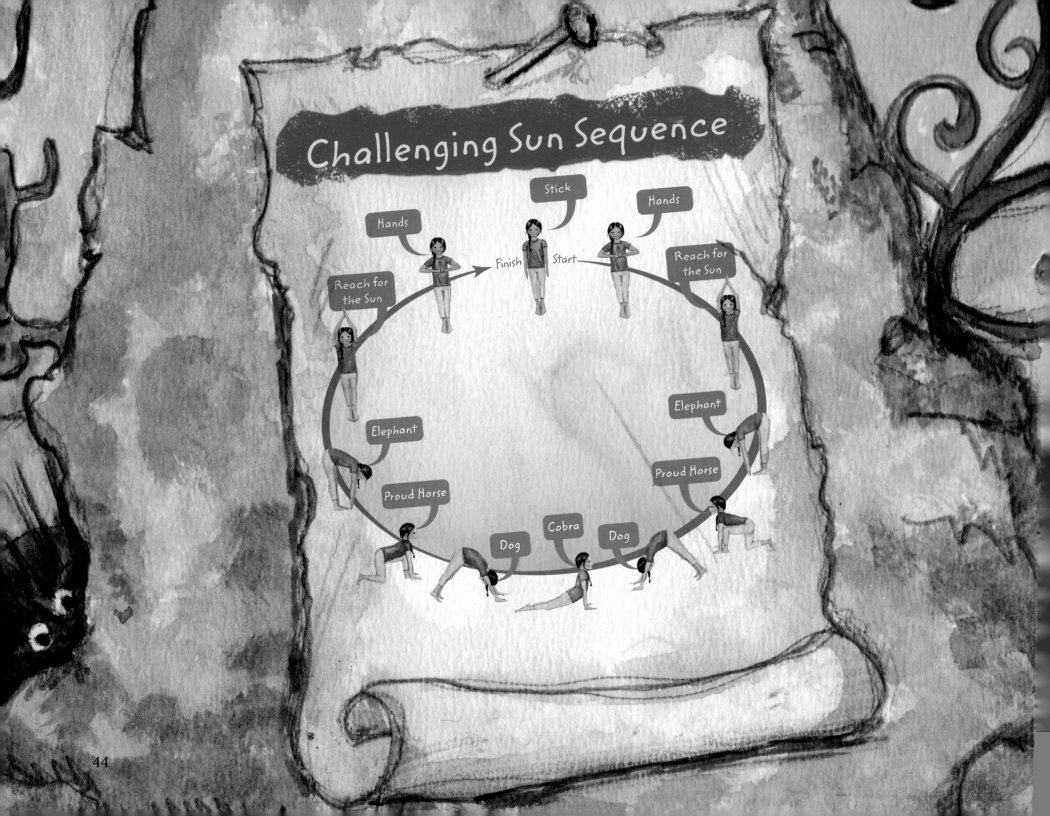

Toddler and Junior said and copied every move. Even though they were a little nervous about attempting a more challenging sequence, they were able to bend and twist well. They were so happy. In fact, they were so happy they asked if they could do it again.

"Of course," said Seahorse. "Toddler, would you like to lead?"

Toddler stepped up, glanced at the paper nailed to the rock and called out the moves.

This time they both bent further forwards in Elephant, and stretched their legs further back in Proud Horse. Above all, they did their best.

"We remembered what you said how it's not very often we see the Sun, living here among the coral, and that if it wasn't for the Sun none of us would be here. So when we do the Sun Sequence we remind ourselves that the Sun is special and maybe a little bit magical," said the Starfish Brothers.

"Which is why," they continued, "when we think about the Sun Sequence a bright glow appears above our heads."

"Thank you and goodbye," said the Starfish Brothers, as they glided silently and easily across the seabed.

Seahorse watched them disappear over the horizon, until all that was left was a brilliant glow above their heads.

A wide smile swept across her face as she glided easily in and out of the coral. Seahorse was happy and ready to deal with whatever the sea-day had to bring. She thought to herself, "Who else can I help today?"

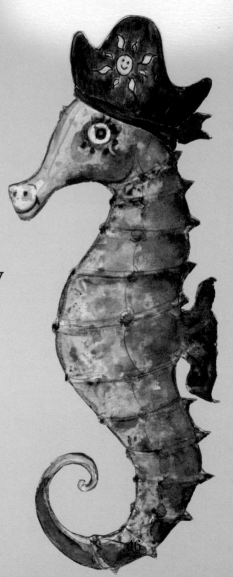

The Sequences in More Detail

The Starfish Brothers: Sun Sequence

This sequence can be used in a variety of situations. I use it with Nursery Children, Reception and Year I in mainstream primary schools in the UK. However, I have also used it with older classes where there may be a child or children who would find the Starfish Brothers Return sequence too demanding. Here is a case study that will help explain.

CASE STUDY: 'TANIA'

'Tania' attends a primary school where I have been teaching for many years. She is a Year I child from Russia who suffers from cerebral palsy. This makes standing and moving around difficult without her walking frame. Her school life has been further challenged because English was not her first language.

I had been teaching Tania's class for two years before she arrived at the school. They were ready to move on to the challenging sequence. However, that would have been a step too far for Tania, so I decided to stick with the first Starfish Brothers sequence, the reason being that she would benefit from more standing postures.

She didn't like it at first. She was petrified that she would fall over. Her Learning Support Assistant helped her to stand. Each week she grew in confidence until four months down the line, she led the class in the Sequence. Every word was crystal clear; with every movement she pushed herself to the limit, and every second it was obvious she enjoyed practising and leading the sequence.

I have used this sequence with Year 6 children when I deemed it more appropriate than other sequences. This sequence is simple, fun and so easy to remember, which is why I also teach it extensively to children with special needs, especially children with autism and sensory processing disorders.

So the message is…be flexible, and use it appropriately.

Eel: Sun Sequence in Wheelchairs

Eel's Sun Sequence is very special. I developed this specifically for children in wheelchairs who have good upper body movement. I have also used this sequence with children who do not have *any* upper body strength or movement, where an adult can help them through the sequence.

Crab: Sun Sequence in Chairs

This is very much the jewel in my crown when I am teaching children with autism and complex sensory problems. Chairs are an important part of the structure of the lesson in this situation. This is because they are more comfortable for children (and adults) than mats and are certainly more familiar to the children. Therefore pupils will be more at ease, less disruptive and less inclined to 'run'. Chairs are also a reference point during the lesson. For example, children can return to their chairs when they have finished the posture. Placing photos of children on their respective chairs can remind them of where to sit. I would set up the chairs in a circle, ensuring that both pupils and adults are in the circle.

Octopus: Sitting Sun Sequence

Do not be fooled! Octopus is the toughest sequence of the four. This sequence was developed for children who:

- Find standing difficult because of a permanent special need, like cerebral palsy, yet have plenty of upper arm strength.

- Have a temporary problem that makes it difficult for them to stand up, for example an ankle or leg injury.

I also wanted to offer an alternative to the Challenging Sun Sequence that contained a spinal twist as well as several different postures, and that challenged children.

The Starfish Brothers Return: Challenging Sun Sequence

Challenging Sun Sequence is the one that I use the most. It is ideally suited to children from Year 2 to Year 6. That is just a guide, so be flexible. If you think that your reception class are ready to move on from Sun Sequence to Challenging Sequence… go for it.

About the Authors

Michael Chissick has been teaching yoga to children in primary mainstream and special needs schools as part of the integrated school day since 1999. He is a leading specialist in teaching yoga to children with Autistic Spectrum Disorders and continues to train and mentor students who want to teach yoga to children. Michael is happy to give advice and guidance about teaching and training to anyone involved in teaching yoga to children. Contact info@yogaatschool.org.uk or visit the website at www.yogaatschool.org.uk

Sarah Peacock is an illustrator and primary school teacher. Following a first class degree in theatre design, Sarah then completed her teacher training in 2004. Her passion for art and illustration are in abundant evidence around the Hertfordshire primary school where she teaches; enhancing not only the school environment, but also providing inspiration to the children. You can contact Sarah at sarahpeacock30@yahoo.co.uk.

Free Sun Sequence Posters

All five sequences are available *for free* in beautifully coloured A3 posters if you own this book. Simply go to www.yogaatschool.org.uk/seahorse, answer a few easy questions and download your free posters.

Beware: Posters will motivate your children to practise and to reap the rewards of Sun Sequences.